National Audit Office

AF885303

Department of Energy & Climate Change

Early contracts for renewable electricity

Report by the Comptroller and Auditor General

Ordered by the House of Commons
to be printed on 26 June 2014

This report has been prepared under Section 6 of the National Audit Act 1983 for presentation to the House of Commons in accordance with Section 9 of the Act

Amyas Morse
Comptroller and Auditor General
National Audit Office

24 June 2014

HC 172 | £10.00

This report examines the rationale for the FIDeR scheme and the value for money of these early contracts.

10470 06/14 NAO

Contents

The National Audit Office study team consisted of:
George Last, David Howes, Stanley Kwong and Eric Lewis, under the direction of Jill Goldsmith.

This report can be found on the National Audit Office website at www.nao.org.uk

For further information about the National Audit Office please contact:

National Audit Office
Press Office
157–197 Buckingham Palace Road
Victoria
London
SW1W 9SP

Tel: 020 7798 7400

Enquiries: www.nao.org.uk/contact-us

Website: www.nao.org.uk

Twitter: @NAOorguk

Key facts

8

contracts awarded under the Final Investment Decision enabling for Renewables Scheme to: five offshore wind farms, two coal plants converted to biomass, and one biomass-combined heat and power plant

£16.6bn

cost to consumers of these contracts over their lifetime, assuming projects commission on time and at their full capacity (2013-14 prices undiscounted)

5

months minimum acceleration of certainty of support from early contracts relative to first allocation round of the main Contracts for Difference regime

17.7 million megawatt-hours	renewable electricity expected from these eight projects in 2020 if they reach their target capacity, before adjusting for transmission losses
324 million megawatt-hours	Department's estimate of the UK's total electricity generation in 2020
5 per cent	estimated proportion of total electricity the eight projects awarded contracts will generate in 2020
30 per cent	Department's estimate of the minimum proportion of total electricity required from renewable sources to meet the UK's 2020 renewable energy target
4548 megawatts	renewable generation capacity these projects should provide
£6.9 billion	estimated funds available for all contracts for renewable electricity projects from 2015-16 to 2020-21, including these early contracts (2013-14 prices undiscounted)
£4 billion	estimated cost of support to these eight projects under the Final Investment Decision enabling for Renewables scheme from 2015-16 to 2020-21, assuming projects commission on time and at their full capacity (2013-14 prices undiscounted)
58 per cent	proportion of the estimated funds available for all contracts for renewable electricity projects taken by these eight projects from 2015-16 to 2020-21

Summary

1 The Department of Energy & Climate Change (the Department) implements energy policy, with three main objectives:

- provide a secure energy supply;
- decarbonise the energy supply; and
- ensure affordable energy for consumers.

2 The Department is responsible for achieving UK climate change commitments. The UK is committed under an EU directive to ensuring that 15 per cent of the energy it uses comes from renewable sources by 2020. To meet this commitment the Department estimates that in 2020 at least 30 per cent of UK electricity needs to come from renewable sources. The Climate Change Act 2008 also commits the government to reduce UK greenhouse gas emissions in 2050 by at least 80 per cent from 1990 levels.

3 To help achieve these objectives, the Department has used the Renewables Obligation to encourage investment in renewable generation. The scheme requires electricity suppliers to pay for Renewables Obligation Certificates. These give renewable generators a premium over the wholesale price for each unit of electricity they supply.

4 As part of its plans for electricity market reform the Department is establishing the Contracts for Difference scheme to replace the Renewables Obligation. Contracts for Difference will set a price for the electricity low carbon generators generate (known as the 'strike price'). A newly formed 'Counterparty Body' will pay generators the difference between the market price and the strike price for the electricity they generate, where the strike price is higher. If the market price is higher than the strike price generators will pay the difference to the Counterparty Body. To enable it to make payments, the Counterparty Body is funded by electricity suppliers which may pass their costs on to consumers. The Department expects to award the first contracts under the main Contracts for Difference regime in December 2014. The Renewables Obligation will close to new projects in April 2017.

5 While developing the main Contracts for Difference scheme in 2011, the Department recognised that developers of low carbon electricity plants, particularly of new nuclear power stations, might delay final investment decisions until they could receive a contract in late 2014. It therefore included in the 2012 Energy Bill the potential for the Secretary of State to award early contracts for difference to enable developers to take these final investment decisions as soon as possible.

6 In March 2013, the Department launched a distinct scheme to award early contracts to renewable generation projects at risk of delay. This scheme was called Final Investment Decision enabling for Renewables (FIDeR). The Department received 57 applications for FIDeR and signed contracts with eight projects in May 2014, subject to European Commission state aid approval. Two of the contracts are for power plants converted from burning coal to biomass, five are for offshore wind farms and one is for a purpose built biomass plant providing heat as well as power.

Scope

7 Our audit addresses the value for money of the contracts awarded under the FIDeR scheme. We evaluated the FIDeR scheme on the following criteria:

- Were the Department's rationale and selection of projects, to award contracts, clearly defined and informed by robust evidence?
- How well has the scheme met the Department's objectives, and achieved good value for money for consumers?

Our methodology is set out in Appendix One.

Key findings

8 **The Department's early contracts are part of its transition to a reformed UK electricity market, designed to attract investment in low carbon generation while offering improved value for money and better cost control.** Contracts for difference under the full electricity market reform regime will be available to nuclear and fossil fuel plants with carbon capture and storage as well as renewables. They should offer better value for money than the existing Renewables Obligation, primarily by guaranteeing the price for each unit of electricity generated which should lower financing costs. For industry the change involves transition from automatic entitlement for Renewables Obligation support for eligible projects, to applying for contracts awarded from a set budget. This gives the Department better control over the costs of support. Early contracts are a component of the transition to this reformed electricity market (paragraphs 1.5 to 1.7).

9 **The Department consciously chose to seek applications before deciding how much renewable generation it wanted from early contracts or whether to cap the budget it would allocate to them.** The Department announced its intention to provide transitional support arrangements in 2011. It launched the scheme in March 2013 to identify the projects that industry considered were at risk of an investment hiatus, making clear that it was making no firm commitment as to the scale of the scheme. At this stage the Department was aware that if all projects which had expressed interest were awarded early contracts, this could commit nearly half the available budget for renewables contracts for difference in 2020. The Department did not determine how much capacity it was seeking from the scheme, nor did it set a budget at this stage. It set the budget for the scheme in November 2013 to enable contracts to be given to the top quarter of qualifying projects in each technology (paragraphs 2.5 to 2.9).

10 The early contracts for eight projects have given those developers certainty of support at least five months earlier than under the full Contracts for Difference regime. The Department's rationale for the scheme was to prevent a hiatus in investment in renewable electricity, enabling developers to take significant or final investment decisions ahead of the full Contracts for Difference regime, the timing for which was uncertain. When the Department invited applications in March 2013, it expected to award early contracts in autumn 2013, a year ahead of the first contracts under the full regime. But the Department subsequently delayed awarding early contracts until April 2014. If the European Commission gives state aid approval for early contracts for the eight projects in July 2014, their developers will be certain of consumer funded support at least five months before award of contracts under the first round of the full regime, currently planned for December 2014. Developers' binding applications stated that without early contracts their projects would be cancelled or delayed by at least 12 months and in one case 24 months (paragraphs 3.2 to 3.5).

11 The Department's assessment of applications tested risks of delay or cancellation, prospects of timely delivery, contributions to development of renewable technology, and affordability. The Department reviewed applicants' statements of the risks to their projects if they did not get an early contract. The Department used its own staff and those from the Department for Business, Innovation & Skills and external consultants to score projects on deliverability and contributions to development of renewable technology. The Department's heads of specialism then moderated those scores. The Department's process obliged it to award contracts to all projects it judged eligible and affordable (paragraphs 2.13 to 2.22).

12 We estimate that the early contracts have committed up to £16.6 billion or 58 per cent of the funds available for renewable contracts for difference to 2020-21. This has given the UK's renewables industry greater confidence in the near term but increased the risk of obtaining support for later projects. Early contracts have given certainty of support to a range of projects and investors in offshore wind and biomass. They are likely to have helped secure other projects' progress and supply chain jobs and investment, including Siemens' investment in wind turbine production and installation facilities in Yorkshire, valued at £160 million. They have also proved the commercial viability of contract terms and conditions for major renewables developers. But the scale of the early contracts has increased the risk for later investors of not getting support (paragraphs 3.9 to 3.12).

13 The early contracts support generation which will help meet the UK's 2020 renewable energy targets, but it is not clear that the full scale of these commitments was needed so soon. The early contracts can provide 5 per cent of total electricity in 2020, though developers may reduce their initially planned capacity by up to 36 per cent without penalty. It is possible that the combination of capacity already operating or with planning consent, and early contracts would more than meet the total capacity from wind and biomass conversion that the Department considers necessary by 2020 to meet the renewables target. But this will depend on attrition rates for projects with planning consent. Even had some capacity been lost or delayed because it did not receive an early contract, the Department might still expect to meet its targets (paragraphs 3.6 to 3.8).

14 **The early contracts have been awarded with administratively set strike prices which may provide higher returns than needed to secure the investment.** The Department set the strike prices to align them with the support available under the Renewables Obligation drawing upon independent advice and reduced strike prices for five technologies following public consultation. The Department considered these prices represented value for money because at that stage they were the same prices it expected to set for the full Contracts for Difference regime. However, administratively set prices may be higher than needed because:

- The Department set strike prices for early contracts at a level designed to encourage the investment needed to meet its decarbonisation objectives. Strike prices are set for each technology rather than negotiated with individual projects. They are designed to offer an acceptable return to the most expensive viable project (the marginal project) needed to meet decarbonisation objectives (paragraphs 3.14 to 3.17).
- Developers are likely to progress those projects offering the most promising returns first, so these early projects may well be those that will benefit most from administrative prices (paragraph 3.14). The Department did not ask for information on estimated project costs and returns, for its own evaluation, since it was not setting project-specific strike prices. It sought that information from applicants to enable the European Commission to consider the risk of over-remuneration as part of its 'state aid' review. The Department has not required contract holders to give information about actual costs and returns (paragraph 3.28).
- The Department offered the same strike price to all phases of offshore wind projects, denying consumers the opportunity to share in any benefit for developers as technological innovation reduces costs. Developers of offshore wind projects have stated that they undertake procurement for all phases of a project at the start of the first phase and do not expect to benefit from cost reductions in later phases (paragraph 3.19).
- The Department has not included provisions to clawback a share of any excessive returns in early contracts. It considered that to do so might deter prospective investors (paragraph 3.27).

15 **The Department's decision to award up to £16.6 billion of early contracts without price competition limits the budget available for later allocation rounds that can use price competition.** The Department proceeded with the scheme while recognising that it did not bring a clear monetised benefit and acknowledging that competitive pricing might reveal subsequently that some administratively set strike prices were too high. It considered early contracts would bring wider benefits to the industry; and the contracts were designed to offer better value than the Renewables Obligation. The Department told us it now expects to apply price competition to up to 40 per cent of the total budget for contracts for difference for renewables between now and 2021 (paragraphs 3.31 to 3.33).

16 **The contracts contain provisions that require active management to protect value for money for consumers.** Their design includes provision for adjusting strike prices, validating power output, and reviewing measures of market prices. The Counterparty Body which will manage these contracts is currently being formed. Under a Framework Agreement, the Department will require the Counterparty Body to "seek to maintain investor confidence in the Contracts for Difference regime and minimise costs to the consumer." Active and effective management of these provisions is essential to ensure contract costs are minimised for consumers (paragraphs 3.23 to 3.25).

Conclusion on value for money

17 Early contracts for renewables have helped industry confidence in the near term and the projects they support can make a significant contribution to meeting the UK's 2020 renewable energy target. The contracts themselves are designed to offer better value for money than the Renewables Obligation they replace. But the contracts have been awarded without price competition and with administratively set strike prices which may provide higher returns than needed to secure investment. We are not convinced that it was essential to award so much consumer support to early contracts in order to meet the 2020 renewables target. Awarding so many early contracts of this scale in this way has limited the Department's opportunity to secure better value for money through competition under the full regime which will start to award contracts in December of this year. The value from the early contracts is in part the learning they can deliver to help transition towards a competitive regime for contracts for difference but this value will be lost if the Department does not get competition into place while a substantial part of the funding remains available.

Recommendations

18 **The Department should ensure that it maximises the opportunity for price competition under the Contracts for Difference scheme.** It could do this by dividing the available budget between technologies and commissioning years, so it is likely to be less than demand, and trigger competitive auctions. Where it has good evidence that the continued availability of support under the Renewables Obligation is preventing genuine competition for strike prices, it should consider reducing the availability or level of Renewables Obligation support.

19 **The Department should include clauses in future Contracts to enable it to clawback excessive returns achieved by individual projects.** It should also consider including provision for reducing strike prices for multiphase projects, for example where there is clear evidence of a significant fall in financing, capital or operating costs since the first phase.

20 **The Department should require holders of all contracts for difference – including early contracts – to give information on their actual costs and returns.** This will let the Department judge whether strike prices are giving expected returns, and use clawback provisions where returns exceed set limits.

21 **The Department should get information from developers on how projects which have been awarded early contracts have contributed to developing the renewables industry in the UK.** The Department evaluated developers' applications for an early contract partly against how they contribute to developing renewable industry supply chains, workforce capacity and renewable technology. It plans to collect information from developers as part of its benefits management strategy. It should ensure it assesses how and whether these claims were realised. It can use this information to help evaluate future contract bids.

22 **The Department should ensure the Counterparty Body actively manages contracts to minimise their costs to consumers while meeting its objectives.** The Department should resource the Counterparty Body to review and challenge generators' claims for increases in strike prices, identify opportunities to reduce strike prices, and check metered output and indices of market prices.

Part One

Final Investment Decision enabling for Renewables

1.1 The Department of Energy & Climate Change (the Department) implements energy policy, with three main objectives:

- to provide a secure energy supply;
- to decarbonise the energy supply; and
- to ensure affordable energy for consumers.

1.2 The Department is also responsible for meeting UK climate change commitments. The government is required by an EU directive to get 15 per cent of energy consumed in the UK from renewable sources by 2020, with interim targets of 4.04 per cent across 2011 and 2012, and 10.21 per cent across 2016 and 2017. In the longer term, the government is legally obliged to reduce UK greenhouse gas emissions by at least 80 per cent by 2050 from 1990 levels. The Department has estimated that the UK needs at least 30 per cent of its electricity generation to come from renewable sources by 2020 in order to meet its renewable energy requirement.

1.3 The Renewables Obligation has been the main support scheme to encourage investment in low carbon electricity generation. Since 2002, the Renewables Obligation has given generators a premium for each megawatt hour (MWh) of renewable electricity they generate. Income from the Renewables Obligation offsets the high cost of setting up and running renewable energy plants. The proportion of the UK's electricity generated from renewable sources has increased from 2 per cent in 2002 to nearly 14 per cent in 2013. The UK met its 2011 and 2012 interim target for energy from renewable sources.

1.4 Since 2011, the Department has been developing electricity market reforms to encourage investment in renewable and other low carbon electricity. It is doing this to help the UK to meet its renewable energy and decarbonisation targets, while maintaining supply and controlling costs for consumers. These reforms were enabled in the Energy Act 2013, which made the following changes:

- **Renewables Obligation**
  Closing the Renewables Obligation to new plants commissioning after 31 March 2017. The scheme will continue to pay premiums already committed until 2037.

- **Contracts for Difference**
  Establishing this new scheme to support new low carbon generation projects commissioning from 1 April 2015. The government expects to award its first contracts to renewable generators under this scheme by the end of 2014.

- **Capacity Market**
  Establishing a Capacity Market for support payments from 2018-19 to ensure sufficient generating capacity from non-intermittent electricity sources (such as gas and coal plants) or to ensure major energy users are ready to reduce their demand when necessary so that supply meets demand.

1.5 Contracts for difference offer low carbon electricity generators an agreed price for the electricity they generate (known as the 'strike price'). A government owned Counterparty Body[1] will pay generators the difference between the market price of electricity (known as the 'reference price') and the strike price. If the market price is higher than the strike price, generators must pay the difference back to the Counterparty Body. The Counterparty Body recoups its costs from electricity suppliers. Electricity suppliers may then pass the costs on to consumers. The government has capped the total cost to consumers of contracts for difference by including them within the Levy Control Framework. The Framework caps existing levy-funded schemes including the Renewables Obligation.[2]

1.6 Contracts for difference should be able to attract investment in a wide range of low carbon generation while offering better value for money and cost control than the Renewables Obligation because:

a The contracts will be available to all types of new investments in low carbon technology, that is nuclear power and fossil fuel power stations fitted with carbon capture and storage, as well as renewable electricity.

b The contracts give generators a shorter, 15-year period of support compared to the 20 years under the Renewables Obligation.

1 The Counterparty Body will be formed as 'The Low Carbon Contracts Company'

2 Comptroller and Auditor General, *Department of Energy and Climate Change: The Levy Control Framework*, Session 2013-14, HC 815, National Audit Office, November 2013.

c The contracts should offer better value for money than the existing Renewables Obligation, primarily by guaranteeing the price for each unit of electricity generated which should lower financing costs.

d The Department sets budgets and rules for allocating contracts. It can control the number and scale of projects receiving support, and the costs of that support. This is in contrast to the Renewables Obligation, which supports any project that meets eligibility criteria.

1.7 The Department has valued the benefits of the Contract for Difference scheme at £10.7 billion (discounted, 2012 prices) up to 2030. This is compared to continuing with existing policy instruments only, principally the Renewables Obligation and carbon pricing.

1.8 While developing the main Contracts for Difference scheme in 2011, developers of low carbon electricity plants, including some new nuclear reactors, raised concerns around uncertainty for projects requiring final investment decisions before contarcts were due to be generally available. The Department recognised these concerns in its July 2011 white paper, and announced its willingess to engage with developers to address consequent risks of project delay or cancellation in its December 2011 technical update. It included in the 2012 Energy Bill the potential for the Secretary of State to award early contracts for difference to enable developers to take these final investment decisions as soon as possible. Since 2012, the Department has been negotiating one early contract with the promoters of a new nuclear plant at Hinkley. It also maintained contact with developers of renewable generation projects.

1.9 In March 2013 the Department set up the Final Investment Decision enabling for Renewables (FIDeR) scheme, to mitigate the risk of a delay to investment in renewable energy. The Department received 57 applications for an early contract through the FIDeR scheme. In April 2014, it announced the award of investment contracts that are early contracts for difference, for eight renewable electricity generation projects and signed contracts in May. Two of the contracts are for coal plants to convert to biomass, five are for offshore wind farms and one is for a dedicated biomass plant providing combined heat and power (**Figure 1** overleaf).

1.10 We estimate that the total lifetime cost to consumers of the eight early contracts awarded could be up to £16.6 billion (undiscounted, 2013-14 prices). This is assuming all projects commission at their target commissioning date and at the full capacity stated in their contracts and is based on the Department's assumptions on load factor and wholesale price (**Figure 2** on page 16). The cost of the contracts for consumers depends on:

- the difference between the wholesale electricity price and the contract strike price; and
- the amount of electricity the plants produce.

If the projects achieve their full capacity and commission at the start of their target commissioning window, they will produce 264 million megawatt hours of renewable electricity over their lifetime. So, the cost of support per megawatt hour is £63.

Figure 1

The early renewable electricity generation contracts

The Department awarded contracts to eight projects, commissioning from 2015 to 2019

Projects	Technology	Target commissioning date	Contract term or fixed end date	Capacity developer aims to install (megawatts)	Strike price (£/ megawatt-hour, 2012 prices)	Strike price (£/ megawatt-hour, 2013-14 prices)	Cost of support (£bn, 2013-14 prices)
Teesside Renewable Energy Project	Biomass combined heat and power	31/07/2018	15 years	299	125	129	1.9
Drax 3rd Conversion Unit (Unit #1)	Biomass conversion	01/02/2016	2027	645	105	108	1.7
Lynemouth Power Station	Biomass conversion	31/12/2015	2027	420	105	108	1.1
Beatrice Offshore Wind Farm – Phase 1	Offshore wind	31/03/2018	15 years	280	140	144	1.0
Beatrice Offshore Wind Farm – Phase 2	Offshore wind	31/03/2019	15 years	384	140	144	1.3
Burbo Bank Extension Offshore Wind Farm	Offshore wind	31/03/2017	15 years	258	150	154	1.0
Dudgeon Offshore Wind Farm – Phase 1	Offshore wind	01/03/2017	15 years	90	150	154	0.4
Dudgeon Offshore Wind Farm – Phase 2	Offshore wind	01/08/2017	15 years	210	150	154	0.8
Dudgeon Offshore Wind Farm – Phase 3	Offshore wind	01/10/2017	15 years	102	150	154	0.4
Hornsea 1st GW Offshore Wind Farm – Phase 1	Offshore wind	31/03/2019	15 years	400	140	144	1.4
Hornsea 1st GW Offshore Wind Farm – Phase 2	Offshore wind	31/03/2020	15 years	400	140	144	1.4
Hornsea 1st GW Offshore Wind Farm - Phase 3	Offshore wind	31/03/2021	15 years	400	140	144	1.4
Walney Extension Offshore Wind Farm – Phase 1	Offshore wind	31/03/2017	15 years	330	150	154	1.3
Walney Extension Offshore Wind Farm – Phase 2	Offshore wind	31/03/2018	15 years	330	150	154	1.3
Total				**4,548**			**16.6**

Figure 1 *continued*
The early renewable electricity generation contracts

Administrative strike prices by commissioning date and technology (2012 £/MWh)

	2014-15	2015-16	2016-17	2017-18	2018-19
Biomass conversions	105	105	105	105	105
Dedicated Biomass with CHP	125	125	125	125	125
Offshore wind	155	155	150	140	140

Notes
1 Contracts for the biomass conversion projects are subject to a fixed end date of 2027.
2 The Department published strike prices in 2012 prices, they are shown here in both 2012 and 2013-14 prices adjusted using the consumer prices index.
3 Cost of support is in 2013-14 prices and is undiscounted. Discounted to present (2013-14) values at a discount rate of 3.5 per cent, the cost of support is £11.4 billion.
4 We have calculated the cost of support on the basis of the capacities and target commissioning dates provided by the project developers in their applications to the scheme, using the Department's load factor assumptions and wholesale price projections from the Department's, Electricity Market Reform Delivery Plan central scenario, December 2013.
5 Under the terms of the contracts, projects may deliver less than these capacities and may commission within the 12-month target commissioning window after the target commissioning date. To assess the cost of these projects, the Department has assumed that some projects have a reduced capacity and commission after the target commissioning date. On this basis, the Department's central estimate of the cost of support is £15.4 billion, undiscounted, (£10.3 billion discounted to present values, at a 3.5 per cent discount rate).
6 Data may not sum due to rounding.

Source: Department of Energy & Climate Change

1.11 One of the applicants is also receiving government backing in other forms. The Drax biomass conversion has a loan from the government owned, but independent, Green Investment Bank. Drax also has a UK government guarantee for a £75 million loan to the company. The terms of this other support can take account of the fact that the project has been awarded a contract under the FIDeR scheme. We are reviewing the government's programme for Loan Guarantees with a view to reporting our findings in autumn 2014.

1.12 In this report we address the value for consumers from these early contracts, in particular addressing:

- the scheme rationale and how the Department selected the projects to award early contracts, in Part Two; and
- the outcome of the process compared to the Department's rationale and the resulting value for consumers, in Part Three.

Figure 2
Cost to consumers of the eight early contracts

The total lifetime contract cost to consumers of the eight early contracts awarded could be up to £16.6 billion

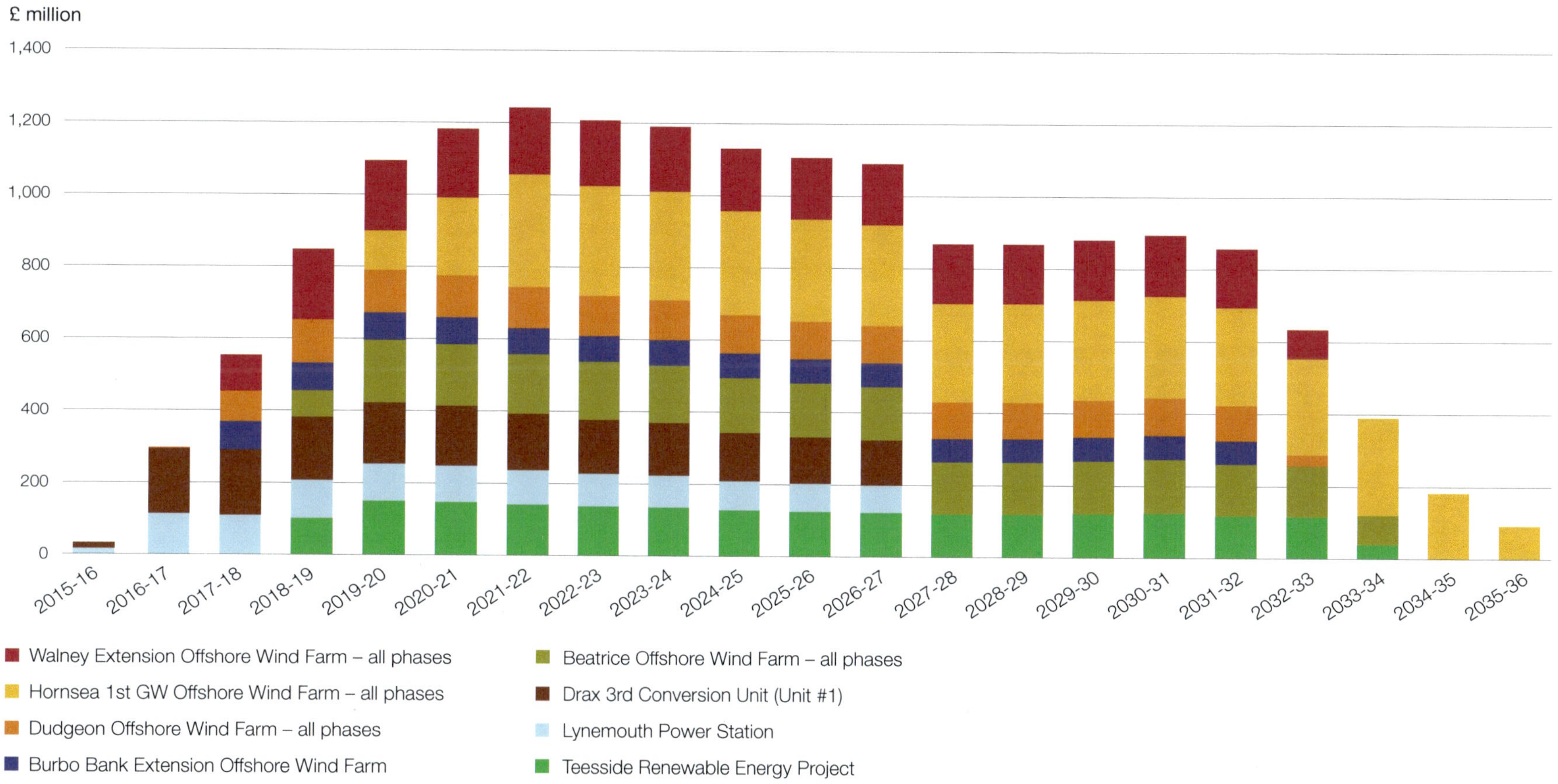

Notes

1 2013-14 prices, undiscounted.

2 Cost of support is in 2013-14 prices and is undiscounted. Discounted to present (2013-14) values at a discount rate of 3.5 per cent, the total cost of support is £11.4 billion.

3 We have calculated the cost of support on the basis of the capacities and target commissioning dates provided by the project developers in their applications to the scheme. We have used the Department's load factor assumptions and wholesale price projections from its Electricity Market Reform Delivery Plan central scenario, December 2013.

4 Under the terms of the contracts, projects may deliver less than these capacities and may commission within the 12-month target commissioning window after the target commissioning date. To assess the cost of these projects, the Department has assumed that some projects have a reduced capacity and commission after the target commissioning date. On this basis, the Department's central estimate of the cost of support is £15.4 billion, undiscounted, (£10.3 billion discounted to present values, at a 3.5 per cent discount rate).

Source: National Audit Office

Part Two

Scheme rationale

2.1 The Department established the Final Investment Decision enabling for Renewables (FIDeR) scheme to enable developers of renewables projects to take final investment decisions which would otherwise be delayed by the uncertainty caused by transition from the Renewables Obligation to the Contracts for Difference regime. It also aimed to provide 'proof of concept' for the Contracts for Difference regime and explore the application of the contracts to a range of renewable energy technologies.

2.2 In this part we look at how the Department:

- assessed the value of early contracts and its business case; and
- addressed its rationale for the scheme in deciding which projects to give contracts to.

Evolving rationale and business case

2.3 From 2011, the Department developed proposals for early contracts for difference for renewable generation projects, based on the business case for the wider programme for Electricity Market Reform. In 2012, the Department developed its case for the Final Investment Decision enabling (FIDe) programme and in November 2012 it published its impact assessment for the FIDe programme, covering proposed early support for new nuclear power, carbon capture and storage projects and renewable electricity. This estimated a net benefit of £2 billion from the impact of the proposed early contract for a nuclear power station. The Department's analysis did not consider the costs and benefits of the two offshore wind farms in isolation from those of the nuclear power plant and so did not identify any distinct benefit from awarding early contracts to the two offshore wind farms.[3] We estimate that the notional costs of support to the two offshore wind farms were £3 billion over the lives of their contracts at 2013 prices.

3 DECC, Impact Assessment: Electricity Market Reform (EMR) Final Investment Decision (FID) Enabling, April 2012, available at: www.parliament.uk/documents/impact-assessments/IA12-033A.pdf.

2.4 Following discussions with 12 developers over the period from 2011, the Department launched the FIDeR scheme in March 2013 for projects that were at significant risk of delay or cancellation if they were required to wait for the main Contracts for Difference regime. It allowed applications for early contracts from those renewable electricity technologies eligible for the Renewables Obligation. The Department told us this was necessary to remain neutral in their approach to different renewable technologies:

- In 2011, the Department had considered there was only a case for awarding contracts to projects that might not commission in time to get Renewables Obligation support. The Department judged that although the Renewables Obligation would continue for projects commissioning before April 2017, projects due to commission shortly before 2017 might not proceed given the risk of slipping beyond eligibility.
- Subsequently, the Department accepted that some projects that could commission well before April 2017 might still be delayed because financiers intended to wait until a contract for difference could underpin revenues. The Department also considered that extending eligibility to such projects might benefit the UK's security of supply. For example, if proposed biomass conversions failed to secure early contracts the unconverted power stations might be forced to close, with a potentially significant impact in the short term on the UK's capacity margins.

2.5 The Department launched the expanded FIDeR scheme in March 2013, with applications to participate required by 1 July 2013 and the intention to award the contracts in autumn 2013. This Phase 1 of the scheme was designed to identify those projects that considered they were at risk of delay. Stakeholders we spoke to confirmed that the intention to award early contracts to this timetable, a year ahead of the Contracts for Difference regime, addressed a genuine risk of investment hiatus. Launching the scheme with wide eligibility criteria raised industry expectations. At this stage the Department was aware that if all projects which had expressed interest in early contracts were awarded them, spend under the scheme could represent 49 per cent of the total available budget for contracts for difference in 2020. But the Department chose not to set a budget for the scheme at this stage. The Department made no firm commitment to industry as to the scale of the scheme, but informed them that it might impose caps on the total funding for early contracts or the budgets made available for different technology types, or both. The Department drew up an outline business case for the scheme in May 2013.

2.6 In June 2013, the Department decided it needed to put back the final award of early contracts to March 2014 as the contract terms to be used for the early contracts (and later for all contracts for difference) were not yet sufficiently well defined. This delay also allowed the Department to align the early contract strike prices with the final strike prices for the main Contracts for Difference regime that it planned to publish in December 2013. The decision to continue with the scheme to this revised timetable was not supported by detailed quantitative economic analysis of the continuing benefits case for the scheme. The Department intended to undertake an economic analysis for its full business case in December 2013. The Department proceeded with the scheme in June 2013 on the grounds that the contracts were needed to prevent a significant hiatus in investment in new renewable electricity generation and there was continuing uncertainty surrounding the timetable for the Contracts for Difference regime, as it depended on achieving Royal Assent of the Energy Bill in December 2013.

2.7 The Major Projects Authority reviewed progress on the scheme in June 2013. Among its findings, it noted that the Department had not yet clarified its success criteria for the scheme, to allow flexibility in its operation. The Authority made recommendations to the Department on clarifying success criteria and on quantifying, measuring and evaluating benefits. In response, the Department developed a plan, showing how it proposes to monitor the impact of projects that receive contracts on the renewables industry and on achieving the UK renewable energy target.

2.8 In value-for-money terms, the decision on what budget to allocate to early contracts was critical. However, the Department did not reach a final decision on this until November 2013. The more money it allocated to early contracts with strike prices set administratively, the less was likely to be available later. The Department set the budget for early contracts high enough to allow the highest ranked 25 per cent of qualifying applicants from each technology to get contracts. This meant three offshore wind projects and one each of onshore wind, biomass conversion and biomass combined heat and power. It set budgets before performing the ranking, so that it did not prejudice which specific projects could be considered affordable. The Department therefore had to assume the top 25 per cent of projects for each technology were also the biggest, or it would risk being unable to fund the largest projects from each technology that had met minimum evaluation thresholds. The Department therefore set the budget for early contracts for the period 2015-16 to 2020-21 at £4.7 billion (2013-14 prices).[4] Based on the applications received it was not possible to spend all of this budget because the Department would not be able to match projects starting in different years precisely to the annual spending limits within the budget and because it expected projects to be delayed.

4 The Department published its budget in 2011-12 prices at £4.5 billion. This is equivalent to £4.7 billion in 2013-14 prices using the consumer price index.

2.9 In November 2013, the Department considered this budget would result in it spending 48 per cent of the funds available within the Levy Control Framework caps for all contracts for difference for renewables to 2020-21, after taking into account the need for a contingency budget. It acknowledged that competitive pricing in the longer term might reveal certain administrative prices had been too high, but also that others may have been set too low. Although the Department expected the Contracts for Difference regime would enable competition in the long run, it considered that initially contracts for less established technologies would be awarded administratively set prices on a first-come first-served basis. It would move to allocation of contracts at fixed times of the year, within fixed budgets, on the basis of price competition where demand for contracts exceeded the available budget.

2.10 The Department's economic analysis at this time showed that awarding early contracts to a potential combination of projects did not have significant monetised costs or benefits compared to alternative scenarios where the scheme did not proceed and projects were delayed or cancelled. The Department's scenarios were for all projects being delayed or all being cancelled. The Department did not consider scenarios with different outcomes by technology or project, nor assess different scales for the scheme and scenarios including future competition to reduce strike prices.

2.11 The Department's investment committee approved the full business case to proceed with the scheme in December 2013. The business case showed there was no clear monetised benefit from the scheme, but identified potential benefits that had not been monetised, which it considered outweighed potential risks to value for money. These were:

- showing that contracts for difference were viable, before the enduring regime;
- reducing industry costs, for example by supporting early supply chain development and by enabling a steady pipeline of projects; and
- minimising the risk of penalties for failing to meet the UK's 2020 renewable energy target and interim targets, by ensuring new capacity could proceed quickly.

Moreover, the Department felt that cancelling the scheme would undermine the confidence of the renewables industry in market support in the UK.

2.12 The Major Projects Authority reviewed the Department's final business case for the FIDeR scheme in January 2014, noting that this business case depended on unquantified benefits. It commended the Department's process for selecting projects and the positive impact on achieving value for money, but noted that there were risks to value for money because of the lack of price competition.

Selecting projects

2.13 The Department selected projects for award of early contracts in three phases (**Figure 3** overleaf):

- Qualification
- Evaluation
- Affordability selection

Qualification

2.14 The Department established qualification criteria that ensured it could reject early speculative applications from projects that did not have detailed plans and could not give supporting evidence. Its qualification process required applicants to demonstrate:

- they had credible plans to start generating electricity by 31 March 2019;
- without an early contract there was a significant risk that the electricity generation to which the contract relates would not occur or would be significantly delayed;
- the project was not already accredited under the Renewables Obligation;
- an expected capacity of 50MW or greater, or in the case of an offshore project, 100MW or greater; and
- the project was located in the UK.

2.15 The Department wanted assurance on the risk of delay or cancellation. It required applicants to show the potential impact of waiting for the full Contracts for Difference regime on the timelines for their critical investment decisions and project commissioning. The Department required a warranted statement from applicants' boards confirming the risk of delay or cancellation. The Department sought further clarification from applicants. But it did not attempt to rank or compare the severity of the risks cited, or the lengths of potential delays to commissioning. The Department told us that to do so would have been too onerous given the number of applicants and the difficulty of treating all applicants equally. Most projects which the Department disqualified did not yet have credible plans or were not eligible technologies. Two applications were disqualified because they did not give convincing evidence that they would face an investment hiatus.

2.16 Applicants with projects commissioning before 2017 could potentially choose between the Renewables Obligation and an early contract. To prove a risk of investment hiatus, they had to explain why support under the Renewables Obligation would lead to delay to or cancellation of the project. Drax sought early contracts for units it planned to convert to biomass. In April 2014, the Department awarded a contract to one unit but disqualified another which had been due to commission first. Drax is currently challenging the Department's decision through a judicial review.

Figure 3

The three-phase project selection process

The Department awarded eight projects from 57 applicants in a three-phase selection process

Phase 1

Qualification (March to June 2013): 57 projects applied, 26 qualified. One project subsequently withdrew.

Phase 2

Evaluation (September to December 2013): the Department scored and ranked detailed applications with minimum thresholds for continued inclusion in the process. Of the 25 remaining projects, 16 met minimum evaluation thresholds.

Phase 3

An affordability selection process (December 2013 to April 2014): The Department assessed how many projects were affordable within its budget. Of the 16, ten were deemed provisionally affordable in December 2013. Before contracts were finally awarded, two onshore wind projects withdrew and one biomass conversion project was disqualified. The Department then awarded a contract to the next highest ranked applicant which was an offshore wind project.

Technology	Applied in Phase 1	Applied for Phase 2	Passed minimum evaluation thresholds	Provisionally affordable in December 2013	Dropped out or disqualified	Awarded contracts
Biomass combined heat and power	5	4	1	1		1
Biomass conversions	6	6	6	3	1	2
Dedicated biomass	3					
Offshore wind	14	12	7	4		5
Onshore wind	18	3	2	2	2	0
Solar Power	7					
Energy from Waste Combined Heat and Power	3					
Tidal range	1					
Total	**57**	**25**	**16**	**10**	**3**	**8**

Source: Department of Energy & Climate Change

Evaluation

2.17 For Phase 2 of the selection process, the Department established evaluation criteria and weighted scores to ensure it selected projects that supported its rationale for the scheme. Projects did not have to compete on price. The Department aimed to select projects against the following criteria:

- **Project deliverability**
  The Department weighted scores to emphasise the projects' technical deliverability (60 per cent of the final score). It also assessed projects' financing plans (15 per cent of the final score). The Department set a minimum threshold for technical deliverability and financing plans. Projects that scored well overall could not proceed unless they scored enough on deliverability because the Department only wanted to take forward projects that were most likely to be completed.

- **Develop renewable technologies**
  The project should help to develop renewable technologies, supply chains and workforce capability (25 per cent of the final score). The Department considered that early deployment of renewable projects, particularly offshore wind, was important to develop the supply chain in the UK and reduce costs of future projects.

2.18 The Department set out for applicants its information requirements for its criteria and evaluation scoring. The Department qualitatively assessed the information and evidence in applicants' submissions. The Department used staff with knowledge of the renewables sector, from their work in the Department's Office for Renewable Energy Deployment and the Department for Business Innovation & Skills, as well as technical advisers from KPMG and Mott MacDonald to assess the projects. It did not draw on other information to assess the plausibility of developers' claims and assumptions. The Department asked for clarifications where it considered it necessary to do so but deliberately did not seek further detail from individual applicants to ensure the process remained fair across all applicants. Stakeholders we spoke to confirmed that the Department did not undertake any additional due diligence on the submissions and in some cases were surprised the Department did not specify more precisely the detailed evidence they required.

2.19 To mitigate the risk of scoring the quality of the applicants' submissions subjectively, each project was scored by two assessors and then moderated. The Department's heads of specialism individually moderated the scores for commercial, technical and industry issues, and re-examined any borderline judgements. We found the assessors and moderators scored consistently and, where there were differences, the Department could give a rationale for the score after moderation.

Affordability selection

2.20 The Department established a technology rule for its affordability selection process to ensure that there was at least one project of each technology type in the process. With the budget set high enough to award contracts to several but not all projects, awarding contracts on ranking alone may have limited support to only one technology type. The Department wanted to give early contracts to more than one type of renewable electricity technology. This was to meet its objective to help develop a range of renewable technologies and enhance industry confidence.

2.21 Applying an affordability selection rule within technologies risked subverting the Department's evaluation process. In principle, the technology selection rule meant lower-scoring projects in one technology could have received a contract before other higher scoring (but unaffordable) projects of a different technology. However, qualifying projects that scored best in the evaluation exercise have all received contracts.

2.22 In December 2013, the Department assessed affordability against its budget. To calculate the cost of support to individual projects, it used its own, lower, estimates for the capacity of four of the sixteen projects which met minimum evaluation criteria rather than the capacity as stated by the developers. It considered this approach provided a realistic upper estimate of costs. After the Department published its list of ten projects which were provisionally affordable in December 2013, two projects withdrew from the process and one was disqualified (Figure 3). The Department estimated that this would leave a total of £1.4 billion of its £4.7 billion budget for early contracts from 2015-16 to 2020-21 unspent, with around £170 million unspent in 2020-21. In line with its published budget allocation process, the Department proceeded to award an additional early contract to the next highest ranked project. This project cost around £420 million from 2015-16 to 2020-21 and took up the £170 million remaining in 2020-21, increasing the number of offshore wind projects supported through the FIDeR scheme from four to five.

Part Three

Outcome of the process

3.1 In this part we address the potential outturn from the early contracts against the range of the Department's objectives. In particular we examine how far the early contracts have:

- avoided an investment hiatus in renewables;
- minimised the risk of missing the 2020 renewable energy target;
- supported industry confidence; and
- achieved value for consumers.

We also compare early contracts with the full Contract for Difference regime.

Avoiding an investment hiatus

3.2 The Department formally launched the FIDeR scheme in March 2013, expecting to award contracts a year earlier than under the main Contracts for Difference regime and so reduce a hiatus in investment in advance of the new arrangements. Developers have continued to invest since December 2011 and successful FIDeR projects will hold valid contracts at least five months ahead of the earliest date possible under the full Contracts for Difference regime. The European Commission is currently considering whether contracts for difference, and individual early contracts, are compatible with EU state aid rules. A decision may be made shortly. The Department currently plans to award the first contracts under the Contracts for Difference regime in December 2014, assuming it can secure European Commission state aid approval and get the necessary secondary legislation in place in time (**Figure 4** overleaf).

Figure 4

The timetable for award of early contracts

The FIDeR scheme has given developers certainty of support at least five months earlier than under the main Contracts for Difference regime

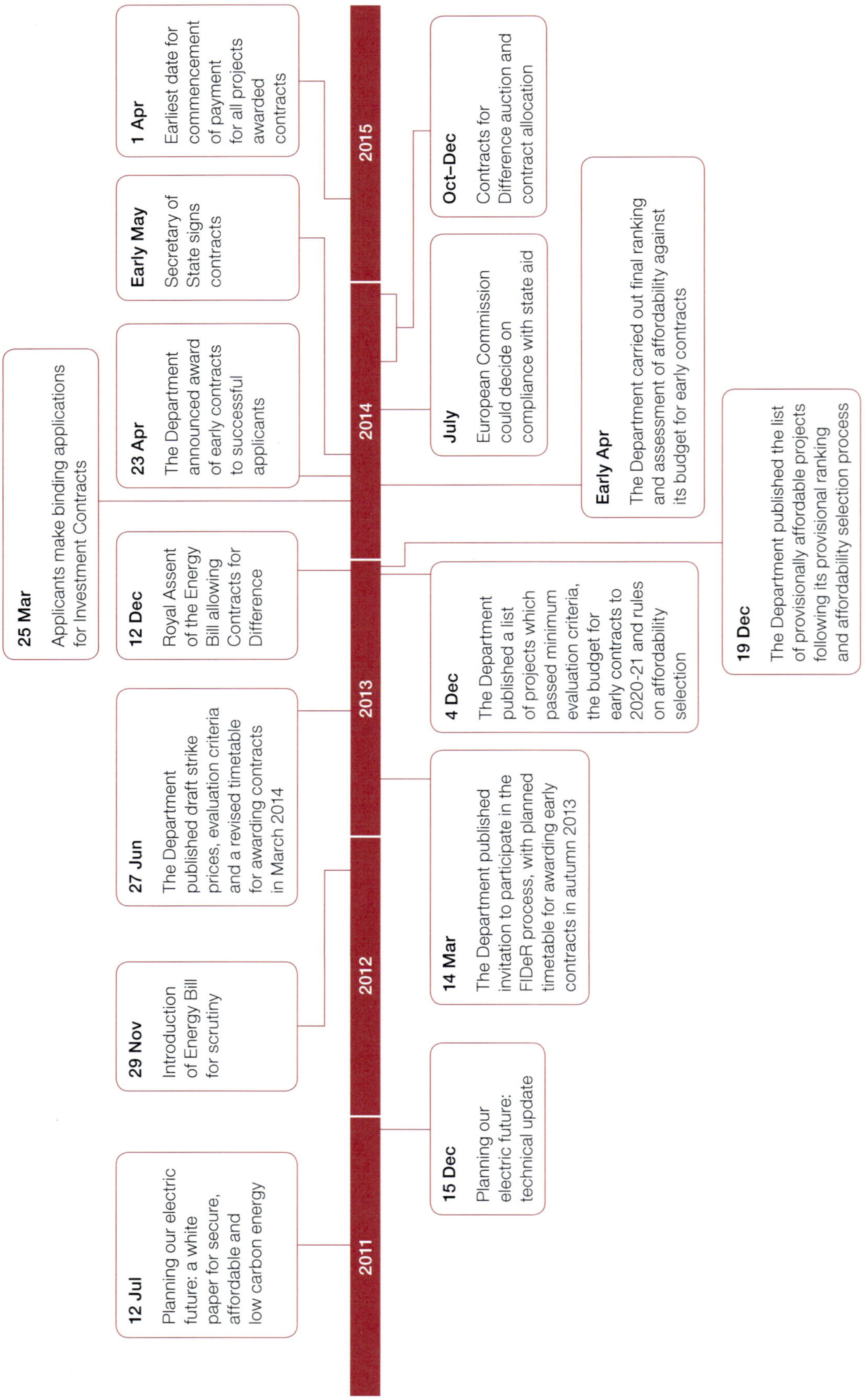

Source: National Audit Office

3.3 The Department's process aimed to give contracts only to projects which would otherwise have been significantly delayed or potentially cancelled. Developers firmed up their expected project commissioning dates as the process progressed and the Department confirmed its contract terms for the early contracts and full Contracts for Difference regime. The commissioning dates identified by applicants in their qualification submissions were later than the target commissioning dates in the binding submissions for three of the projects awarded contracts (**Figure 5** overleaf). Where applicants' binding target commissioning dates are later than in the qualification phase, this could be a reflection of their reassessment of their project timetable or the impact of delays to the contract selection process.

3.4 Three of the offshore wind projects receiving early contracts are yet to receive planning consent, adding a further outstanding milestone to their decision-making and investment paths. The Department scored projects more highly where they had planning consent but did not disqualify those without it. The Department considered it appropriate to award contracts in advance of planning consent to avoid hiatus on offshore wind projects. It confirmed in August 2013 that planning consent would be a pre-requirement for the main Contracts for Difference regime. This gave projects an additional incentive to confirm their application for an early contract.

3.5 Developers' final binding applications for the contracts stated for two projects that they would have been at significant risk of cancellation, for five projects that they would have been delayed by at least 12 months, and for one offshore wind project without planning consent that it would be delayed by 24 months. The Department considers that applicants' assessment of the delay avoided is greater than five months because the scheme encouraged developers to progress projects through design, approval, and procurement commitments earlier than would have been possible had they waited for the full Contracts for Difference regime.

The 2020 renewable energy target

3.6 The contracts will provide generation which will be commissioned before 2020 and will help meet the 2020 renewable energy targets. To meet the target, the Department estimated in December 2013, that approximately 110 million megawatt-hours of renewable electricity, just over 30 per cent, of electricity must come from renewable sources. This is from an installed capacity of around 43,000 megawatts. Renewable generation in the UK in 2013 was some 50 million megawatt-hours, equivalent to nearly 14 per cent of total generation, from an installed capacity of around 19,500 megawatts. The Department expects the eight selected projects to give an extra 4,548 megawatts in capacity and generate 17.7 million megawatt-hours in 2020. This will add 5 per cent to the proportion of the UK's electricity generation from renewable sources. (**Figure 6** on page 29).

Figure 5
Commissioning dates

Commissioning dates for three of the eight selected projects are earlier than they were in applicants' phase 1 submissions in early 2013

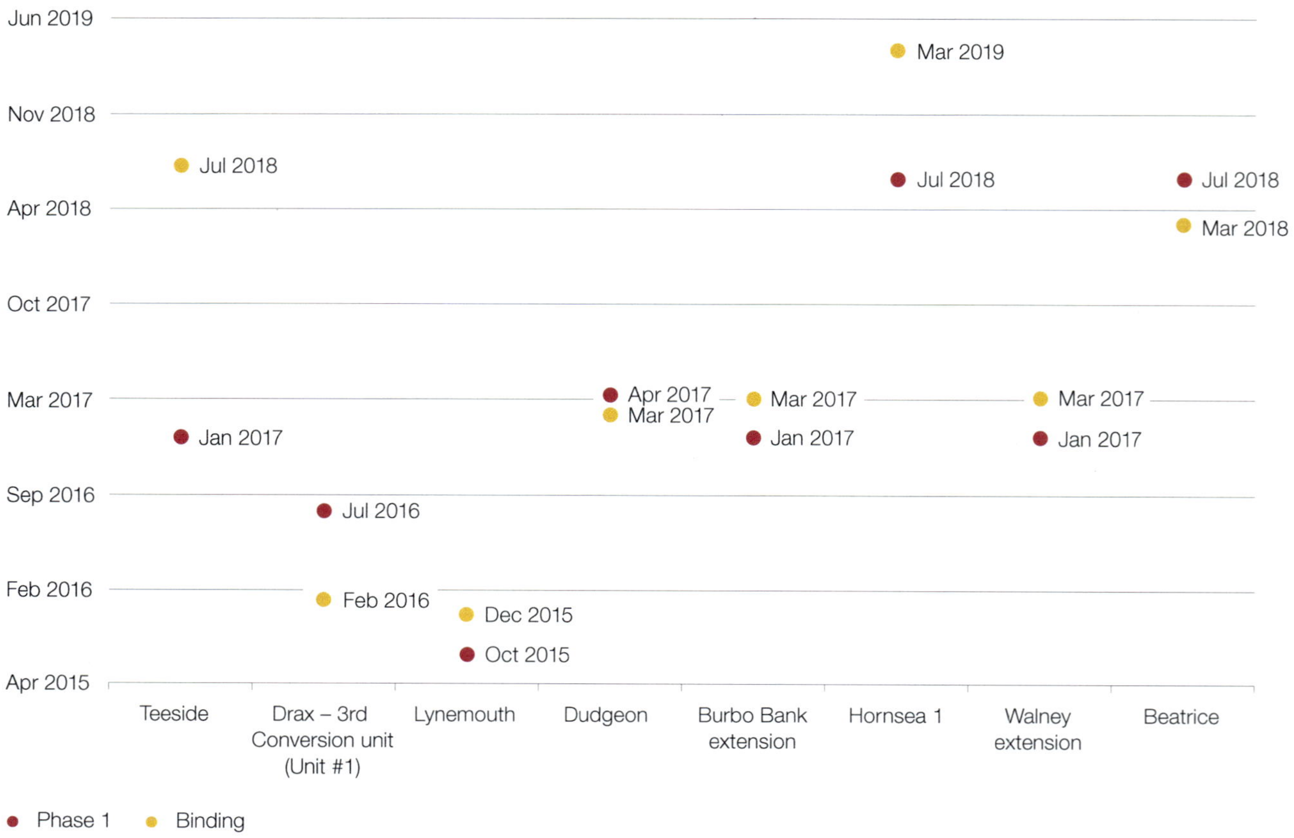

Description	Technology	Expected commissioning date at Phase 1 of the FIDeR process	Target commissioning date as per developers' binding submissions
Teesside	Biomass CHP	Jan 2017 to Mar 2017	31 Jul 2018
Drax – 3rd Conversion Unit (Unit #1)	Biomass conversion	Jul 2016	1 Feb 2016
Lynemouth	Biomass conversion	Oct 2015	31 Dec 2015
Dudgeon	Offshore wind	Apr 2017 to Mar 2018	1 Mar 2017
Burbo Bank extension	Offshore wind	Jan 2017 to Mar 2017	31 Mar 2017
Hornsea 1	Offshore wind	Jul 2018 to Sep 2018	31 Mar 2019
Walney extension	Offshore wind	Jan 2017 to Mar 2017	31 Mar 2017
Beatrice	Offshore wind	Jul 2018 to Sep 2018	31 Mar 2018

Notes

1 For the purposes of this graphic, we have shown the earlier date of the ranges supplied in developers' submissions at the qualification phase of the FIDeR scheme.

2 Target commissioning dates are the first day of a 'target commissioning window' which runs for a year, so projects may well commission later than the target commissioning date.

Source: National Audit Office

Figure 6

UK Renewable energy generation to 2020 by FIDeR projects

The selected FIDeR projects could contribute 5 per cent of total UK generation in 2020

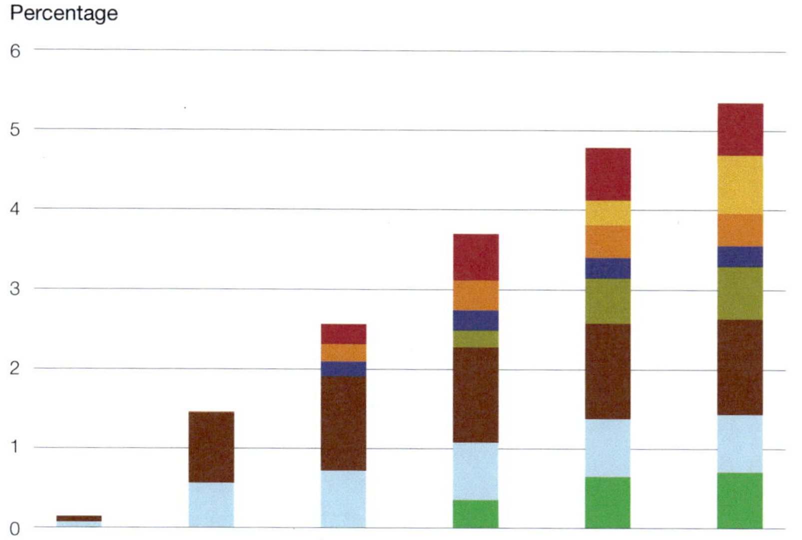

	2015	2016	2017	2018	2019	2020
Walney Extension Offshore Wind Farm – all phases	0.00	0.00	0.25	0.58	0.66	0.66
Hornsea 1st GW Offshore Wind Farm – all phases	0.00	0.00	0.00	0.00	0.32	0.73
Dudgeon Offshore Wind Farm – all phases	0.00	0.01	0.21	0.37	0.40	0.40
Burbo Bank Extension Offshore Wind Farm	0.00	0.00	0.19	0.26	0.26	0.26
Beatrice Offshore Wind Farm – all phases	0.00	0.00	0.00	0.21	0.57	0.66
Drax 3rd Conversion Unit (Unit #1)	0.07	0.88	1.18	1.20	1.20	1.20
Lynemouth Power Station	0.07	0.57	0.72	0.72	0.72	0.72
Teesside Renewable Energy Project	0.00	0.00	0.00	0.36	0.66	0.71

Notes

1 Assuming projects commission at their target commissioning dates and at their full capacity.

2 Percentage calculated before adjusting for transmission losses.

3 Data is in calendar, not financial, years.

Source: National Audit Office

3.7 It is not clear that the full scale of these commitments was needed so soon. Even if some capacity had been lost because projects did not receive an early contract, the Department might still have been able to meet its targets:

- In its December 2013 Electricity Market Reform delivery plan, the Department estimated that it needed 43,000 MW renewable electricity in total, including some 25,600 MW capacity from onshore wind, offshore wind, and biomass to meet the target in 2020.
- The Department's information on the pipeline of renewable generation projects shows that the renewables industry has grown strongly, although this does not provide a clear indication of commissioning dates. Together with renewable electricity capacity in operation and under construction and with planning consent the early contracts could deliver 29,300 MW capacity for onshore wind, offshore wind and biomass. Based on its latest estimates of historic attrition rates, the Department expects 30 per cent of onshore wind projects with planning consent and awaiting construction will not proceed to commissioning.[5] Applying this rate to onshore wind, offshore wind and biomass projects with planning consent but awaiting construction could reduce the capacity to 25,800 MW. Including proposed projects which do not currently have planning consent, including those supported with early contracts, could deliver total capacity of 48,400 MW. Applying a 65 per cent attrition rate for projects not yet having planning consent could reduce this capacity to 32,500 MW (**Figure 7**).
- The Department expects to be able to encourage additional capacity to 2020 within its Levy Control Framework caps, and that competition will drive down strike prices for onshore wind and solar power below the administrative prices it has published.

5 Historic attrition rates may not accurately reflect attrition rates in the years between now and 2020.

Figure 7

Operational and planned electricity generation capacity from offshore wind, onshore wind and biomass plants in April 2014

There should be sufficient generation capacity in the pipeline to meet the 2020 renewables target

	Projects with planning consent					Projects awaiting planning consent			
Technology (MW)	Operational	Under construction	Awaiting construction	Total capacity with planning consent or operational	Supported through FIDeR	Capacity awaiting planning consent	Supported through FIDeR	Total capacity operational or in the planning pipeline	Deployment in 2020: EMR Delivery Plan, December 2013 (incl small scale generation)
Onshore wind	7,406	1,539	5,226	14,170	0	6,432	0	20,603	11,700 – 14,100
Offshore wind	3,969	1,401	4,152	9,522	1,066	12,338	2,118	21,860	8,100 – 15,000
Biomass	3,136	268	2,217	5,621	1,364	299	0	5,919	2,500 – 4,600
Total for onshore wind, offshore wind and Biomass	14,511	3,208	11,594	29,313	2,430	19,069	2,118	48,381	22,300 – 33,700 25,600 (deployment in Electricity Market Reform Delivery Plan reference case)

Notes

1 We have taken deployment ranges in 2020 from the Department's modelling for its Electricitiy Market Reform final delivery plan, December 2013. The single total is from the reference case developed for this modelling which is Scenario 1 in the delivery plan.

2 Other data is taken from the Department's Renewables Energy Planning Database, Progress datasheet, May 2014.

3 Biomass includes biomass conversion and biomass combined heat and power.

4 Not all of this capacity will be installed as projects awaiting construction may not be built and projects may not receive planning consent. The rate of attrition will vary from technology to technology.

5 Planning pipelines do not take into account sensitivities such as the possible impact of policy developments or changes in financial support rates.

6 Data may not sum due to rounding.

Source: Department of Energy & Climate Change

3.8 There remains uncertainty over the actual contribution of the projects awarded early contracts to the UK's renewable energy targets. At the project planning stage of renewable electricity investments there is always some uncertainty around the time required to construct a plant and its final capacity once commissioned. Through the scheme the Department consulted applicants and industry more widely on the terms for the contracts to encourage developers to deliver in line with contractual commitments. The resulting terms ensure that consumers only pay for the energy actually generated and penalise developers if they do not meet their commitments on the timing for and scale of plant being commissioned. However, they do not fully mitigate the risks to the government from tying up consumer funding for projects which do not proceed:

- **Penalties**
  If the generator commissions after the last day of the target commissioning window this reduces the period of support under the contract. If delivery slips beyond a 'long-stop' date one or two years after close of the target commissioning window, the Counterparty Body can terminate the contract without compensation. The Counterparty Body may also withdraw the contract if the developer does not spend a specified amount or meet other specific commitments by a milestone delivery date. But there is no penalty beyond loss of the contract for failure to deliver.

- **Reducing capacity**
  Generators can reduce their planned installed capacity by up to 25 per cent before their agreed milestone delivery date, without losing their contract. Thereafter generators must deliver 85 per cent of that revised capacity or lose the contract. Generators can reduce their planned installed capacity further without penalty if there is an unforeseen geological condition or physical constraint which renders installation of the planned capacity uneconomic, provided they have acted to a reasonable and prudent standard in developing the project. Overall the definition of events allowing a change of capacity is broad. Even without such a change, the final amount commissioned could be only 64 per cent of that planned at contract award without losing the contract.

Impacts on industry confidence

3.9 The FIDeR scheme has helped the Department define the detailed conditions and terms of a contract for difference and shown industry that the concept of a contract for difference is workable in practice. The Department considers this proof that contracts for difference are workable is important for maintaining investor confidence in the continued availability of government support for renewable projects in the UK.

3.10 The Department expects these early contracts to benefit the renewables industry and to have helped secure earlier some supply chain jobs and investment associated with the supported projects. As part of their submissions, projects have shown how they will help to develop renewable electricity technology, their supply chains and their workforce capacity. Siemens told us that their £160 million investment decision for developing wind turbine production and installation facilities in Yorkshire was helped by the contracts provided under FIDeR scheme. Statkraft told the Department they had invested in design studies and geotechnical surveys in advance of receiving a final contract because the FIDeR scheme had given them the confidence that award of a contract was likely.

3.11 By using a high proportion of the latest estimates of the available Levy Control Framework budget, early contracts may reduce industry confidence in getting support later in the decade. Stakeholders we spoke to noted that the constrained funds available for other renewable contracts for difference increased the allocation risk for future projects. Assuming these projects commission at their target commissioning date and at their full capacity, they will cost £4 billion to 2020-21, 58 per cent of the £6.9 billion we estimate is available for all renewable contracts for difference. In 2020-21, these projects will cost £1.2 billion, 65 per cent of the £1.8 billion available in that year (**Figure 8** overleaf).[6] The amount of funding available for new contracts will depend on the Department's controls on spending on other schemes. For example, the cost of the Renewables Obligation could increase if large numbers of renewable generation projects seek to accredit before it closes in 2017. The budget available for contracts for difference for renewables also depends on the strike prices agreed and the actual commissioning date for non-renewable projects, such as carbon capture and storage.

6 Cost data are in 2013-14 prices. The Department considers these eight FIDeR projects may deliver less than the full capacity stated by developers and could commission later than target commissioning dates. On the basis of its adjusted estimates of capacity and commissioning dates, the Department's central estimate of the cost of these contracts between 2015-16 and 2020-21 is £3.2 billion (undiscounted), 47 per cent of the available funds. In 2020-21, the Department's central estimate is that they will cost £1 billion, 57 per cent of the available funds in that year.

Post publication this page was found to contain an error which has been corrected (Please find Published Correction Slip)

Figure 8

Forecast spending on early contracts

Forecast spending on early contracts limits the funding available under the main Contracts for Difference regime

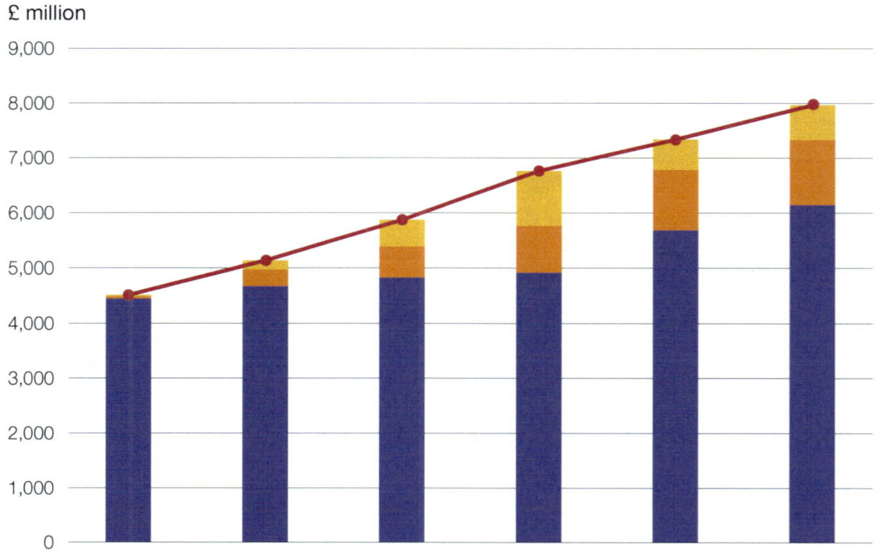

	2015-16	2016-17	2017-18	2018-19	2019-20	2020-21
Estimated funds available for other renewable contracts for difference	29	167	486	994	555	634
Estimated FIDeR cost (using projects' full capacity estimates and target commissioning dates)	31	296	553	848	1,093	1,182
Other budgets (Renewables Obligation, small scale Feed-in Tariffs, contracts for Difference for non-renewable technologies, contingency)	4,448	4,675	4,833	4,921	5,691	6,151
LCF cap	4,508	5,137	5,871	6,762	7,339	7,968

Notes

1 Cost data are in 2013-14 prices, undiscounted.

2 The amount remaining for renewable electricity projects under the main Contracts for Difference regime is uncertain and the Department has yet to set its budgets for this regime.

3 The cost of the Renewables Obligation could increase significantly if several new projects, including those unsuccessful in the FIDeR scheme, seek accreditation before it closes to new accreditations in April 2017. This would further reduce the budget for Contracts for Difference.

4 We have calculated the cost of FIDeR on the basis of the capacities and target commissioning dates provided by the project developers in their applications to the scheme, using the Department's wholesale price projections from the Department's, EMR Delivery Plan central scenario, December 2013.

5 Under the terms of the contracts, projects may deliver less than these capacities and may commission within the 12-month target commissioning window after the target commissioning date. To assess the cost of these projects, the Department has assumed that some projects have a reduced capacity and commission after the target commissioning date. On this basis, the Department's central estimate of the cost of these contracts between 2015-16 and 2020-21 is £3.2 billion (undiscounted), 47 per cent of the available funds. In 2020-21, the Department's central estimate is that they will cost £1 billion, 57 per cent of the available funds in that year.

Source: Department of Energy & Climate Change

3.12 At the Budget 2014, the government decided to cap the carbon price floor from 2016-17 to 2019-20. The higher the carbon price floor, the higher the tax paid on fossil fuels used for electricity generation. Capping it means that wholesale electricity prices are lower than if the carbon price had been allowed to rise in line with original plans. This is turn means difference payments under contracts for difference are higher. This has increased the risk that the Department may not be able to allocate enough contracts for difference to support investment to meet the renewables target within the Levy Control Framework caps. Using the Department's data, we estimate that capping the carbon price floor will add £225 million to the cost of these early contracts between 2016-17 and 2020-21, of which around £85 million is in 2020-21. The Department has stated that it will maintain the 'buying power' of the Levy Control Framework. To do this, it is increasing its Levy Control Framework budget by around £170 million in 2020-21 (2013-14 prices), but is not altering the overall cap. So it is reducing the contingency available to absorb other cost increases within the Levy Control Framework.

Early contracts' value for consumers

3.13 These contracts could cost consumers up to £16.6 billion to 2036 (2013-14 prices). The main drivers of the contract cost for consumers are the strike price, the reference price (which is the wholesale price) and the quantity of electricity produced. Where the strike price is higher than the reference price, the Counterparty Body pays the generator the difference between the strike price and the reference price for each unit of electricity it contributes to grid output. If the reference price exceeds the strike price, the generator pays the difference to the Counterparty Body. Given the long duration of these contracts, there are risks to public value if the terms of the contracts overpay developers. We have identified risks to public value from the contracts arising from:

- how the Department set strike prices;
- inflation indexation of strike prices;
- specifying the reference price;
- allowing for changes in costs;
- specifying the output; and
- returns to investors.

Strike price setting

3.14 The Department set the strike prices for early contracts and later contracts for difference to ensure that plant with costs just low enough to yield the required rate of return and still be viable (the marginal plant) under the Renewables Obligation would also be the marginal plant under the Contracts for Difference regime.

3.15 The Department set levels of support under the Renewables Obligation after its 2012 review of the number ('bands') of Renewables Obligation Certificates (ROCs) for each renewables technology. The number of ROCs per megawatt-hour of electricity from each technology was designed to bring forward a mix of projects sufficient to meet the 2020 renewable energy target. To achieve this, the Department used estimates, for each technology, of:

- the range of capital and operating costs per megawatt of generating capacity;
- the rate of return required by investors (the 'hurdle rate') to proceed with a project; and
- the actual electricity a plant generated as a proportion of its maximum capacity (its load factor).

The Department used these estimates to model what plants would be viable and hence how much renewable electricity capacity might be deployed under different levels of Renewables Obligation support.

3.16 In setting the strike prices the Department assumed that hurdle rates would be lower under contracts for difference because they remove wholesale price risk (**Figure 9**). This reflected the Department's view that contracts for difference would be better value for money compared to the Renewables Obligation. The removal of wholesale price risk would reduce financing costs and allow the bidding generator to sell their electricity to electricity suppliers through long-term power purchase agreements at more favourable prices. The Department tested different levels of strike prices and chose those that gave the returns investors might need to support the marginal plant for each technology. It set lower strike prices for some technologies for projects commissioning after the Renewables Obligation closed, to account for potential cost reductions.

3.17 The Department sought independent advice on the analysis underpinning its strike prices, from its panel of technical experts and from consultants NERA Economic Consulting. It also ran a consultation between July and December 2013 to obtain views from other stakeholders on whether the strike prices it proposed were appropriate. As a result of this process the Department reduced its strike prices for five technologies.[7]

7 Onshore wind, large-scale solar, sewage gas, landfill gas, energy from waste with combined heat and power.

Figure 9
Hurdle Rate Comparison

Hurdle rates for offshore wind and biomass conversion projects with a contract for difference are expected to be lower than under the Renewables Obligation

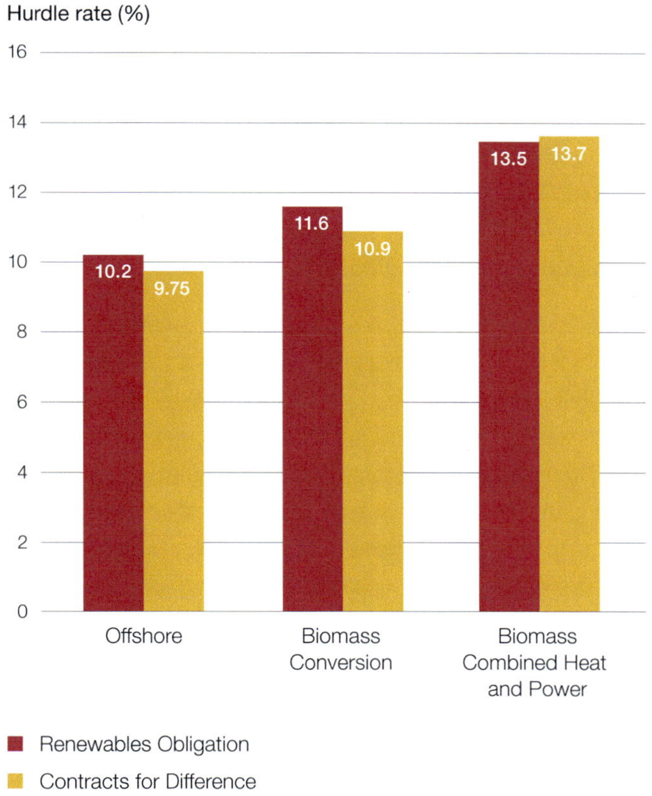

Note

1 Hurdle rates are estimated in pre-tax real, 2012 prices.

Source: Department of Energy & Climate Change

3.18 The Department may nonetheless not have accurately estimated the value of a contract for difference over the Renewables Obligation in setting its strike prices. The hurdle rates the Department assumed to set strike prices may be higher than the rates investors required. While noting the difficulty of drawing straightforward comparisons with the UK and the different risk sharing arrangements between governments and investors, the 2013 NERA analysis for the Department showed that investors in similar renewable electricity projects elsewhere in Europe had accepted lower returns.[8] Also, the share price of Drax rose significantly when the Department shortlisted it for early contracts to convert two of its units to biomass. When the Department did not offer one of those units an early contract, the Drax share price fell sharply, even though the unit could still benefit from Renewables Obligation support. This suggests the market valued early contracts for difference more than Renewables Obligation support for this plant, although further factors may also have contributed.

3.19 The Department has set the strike prices awarded in these contracts depending on the year in which the project is expected to commission. For four of the offshore wind projects it has agreed this price for all of their phases. The Department expects technology costs to fall, so has set lower strike prices for projects commissioning in later years. By agreeing multiphase contracts with strike prices for the first phase the Department prevents the consumer from benefiting from falling costs, which may happen through technology development on the projects in later phases. If the reduced strike prices for later phases were applied to the four multiphase offshore wind projects this would reduce costs to consumers by around £325 million.[9] Developers of offshore wind projects seek contractual certainty for all phases before they will commit to a project. They told us that they undertake procurement for all phases at the start of the first phase and do not expect to realise cost reductions over the course of their projects.

Inflation indexation of strike prices

3.20 The FIDeR contracts provide that strike prices will be increased in line with inflation, as measured by the Consumer Price Index (CPI). The contracts do not allow for changes in the strike price to reduce costs to consumers, if developers benefit from this protection. The Department allowed inflation indexation because consumers are thought to be better placed to absorb the impact of high inflation than generators. Yet generators could fix the cost of their debt repayments, especially once plant is complete and commissioned, and these debt costs will form a significant share of total project costs. There is no option in these early contracts for difference for renewables to de-index part of the strike price (and recalculate the initial strike price to maintain the project's rate of return) if the developer is able to finance the project using fixed rate debt. Strike prices would need to be higher initially, if they were not fully indexed. That could nevertheless be better value for money for consumers over the life of the contract.

8 NERA Economic Consulting, *Changes in Hurdle Rates for Low Carbon Generation Technologies due to the Shift from the UK Renewables obligation to a Contracts for Difference* (December 2013), p.101ff.

9 To estimate these figures, we have applied the £140 strike price to those phases of offshore wind projects with a target commissioning date on or after 1 April 2017.

Reference prices

3.21 The support for generators will be the difference between the strike price and the wholesale price. Generators may sell their electricity for more or less than the 'reference price' used to measure the wholesale price. The contracts set the reference price using trading indices. The Department used day-ahead electricity markets for intermittent generation (for example wind), and season-ahead markets for baseload generation (for example biomass). Generators will bear any loss or gain from the reference price being different from the price they get for their electricity.

3.22 Poor liquidity in the wholesale electricity market means there is a risk that generators could manipulate the reference price. Ofgem has found that wholesale electricity market liquidity is poor, particularly for products traded long before they will be supplied (for example for future months or seasons). Individual trades in the season-ahead reference market used for baseload contracts could influence the reference price. Manipulation might occur if, for example, a generator sold its electricity through the market to an associated company at an artificially low rate. This could depress the reference price and increase the difference payments funded by consumers. And the associated company might keep the profit rather than pass it on to customers. This risk is mitigated by Ofgem's ability to monitor and investigate trades and take action if they believe market abuse has occurred. The Department has sought advice on this risk from KPMG in relation to the proposed contract for difference for a Hinkley Point C nuclear power plant and considers it not to be significant.

Cost

3.23 Providing price support under contracts for difference means the developer generally bears the opportunities (and risks) of their costs being lower (or higher) than those assumed in setting the strike price. However, the FIDeR contracts provide for the Department to adjust strike prices or pay a lump sum if costs change because of certain changes in law or regulation which bear distinctly or disproportionately on the developer. Such changes might include, for example, a new statutory health and safety standard affecting storage of fuel for a specific type of biomass plant. Or a new protection requirement for a seabed type, bearing only on the sole offshore wind farm located on that seabed type.

3.24 The contracts say that the generator will bear certain charges from National Grid for balancing supply and demand across the transmission system. They also say that a specified proportion of the generator's output will be lost in transmission as it is transported over the grid. Changes in these balancing charges and transmission losses relative to those assumed at contract award, are passed through to consumers through annual adjustments to strike prices.

3.25 The Counterparty Body will need to actively manage contracts, to ensure claims for increases in strike prices are reasonable, and to identify and apply reductions in strike prices. The Department has progressed its plans for the establishment of the Counterparty Body. It has appointed a Chair, and contract manager and expects to confirm the appointment of the Chief Executive Officer shortly, and is developing a Framework Agreement to set expectations for the roles of the Department and the Counterparty Body and require the Counterparty Body to "seek to maintain investor confidence in the Contracts for Difference regime and minimise costs to the consumer."

Output

3.26 The contracts have extensive provisions to ensure that generators record and report their output, including provisions on validating metering arrangements. The Counterparty Body will need to understand and use its powers under these provisions to protect consumers from paying for more output than is actually provided.

Project returns

3.27 The Department set the strike prices to match the expected returns available to developers under the existing Renewables Obligation scheme. It has not included in the contracts any provision to claw back excessive returns. This is despite developers being able to benefit from the inflation provision and reference price specification. The Department could have included, for example, a cap on the rate of return. It considered that to do so would be impractical because of the requirement for detailed financial due diligence for each project around a contract financial model.

3.28 As part of its normal state aid assessment process, the European Commission will consider the risk of over-remuneration under the UK's proposed contracts for difference, including the early investment contracts. To do so they asked the Department to collect information from developers on their expected returns from the projects receiving early investment contracts. The Department collected this information after it had announced which projects would receive an early contract.

3.29 The Department has not required generators to give the information needed to assess their actual returns. The contracts require generators to give the Counterparty Body the information it needs to perform and report on its obligations under the contracts and in wider law. This does not require generators to give information on the costs, revenues, and returns available to or made by their projects holding contracts for difference. Information on actual returns would be useful in judging the appropriate strike price for new contracts, and the merit of requiring claw back of 'excess' returns in new contracts.

3.30 The Department plans to ask developers for information on their actual contribution to industry or supply chain development for its assessment of the benefits realised by the scheme. However, it has not sought powers within the terms of the contract to require generators to provide this information. Such information would help the Department judge the wider economic benefit of support for renewable generation, including creating jobs in the UK. It could also help identify innovations in manufacture or plant installation, which could lower costs across the industry.

Early contracts and full contracts for difference

3.31 The Renewables Obligation supports all eligible projects. The FIDeR scheme supported the best projects for the same technologies at their given prices within the available budget. The Contracts for Difference regime may introduce price competition and improve value for money. If the Department had not awarded early contracts under the FIDeR scheme the extent to which it could have got equivalent generation under the Contracts for Difference regime for lower cost will depend on whether the Department moves to a competitive regime for contracts for difference.

3.32 When it awarded early contracts the Department did not expect demand and market confidence to allow a move to competitive pricing for all technologies until 2017. For contracts awarded before then, it was envisaging price competition for established technologies (onshore wind and solar) from the first allocation round of the full Contracts for Difference regime in December 2014. For less established technologies (offshore wind and dedicated biomass providing combined heat and power) the Department did not envisage price competition in the first round. The Department had not decided its approach for biomass conversion (**Figure 10** overleaf).

3.33 The Department told us its latest estimates suggest up to 40 per cent of the total budget for contracts for difference for renewables could be available for competitive allocation between now and 2021. This could cover all technologies, representing a significant change in the Department's view of the timing and extent of the opportunity for price competition for renewables support. The estimate is based on latest figures for spending under the Renewable Obligation, latest provisional fossil fuel price projections, and expected rather than maximum spend under early contracts. It also assumes all Levy Control Framework budget is available for spending, with none held back for contingencies. It is subject to fluctuation given the wide range of factors influencing expenditure under the schemes included in the Levy Control Framework.

Figure 10
Contracts for Difference scheme budget pots

In early 2014, the Department was proposing to divide the budget for the Contracts for Difference regime into three pots

Pot 1	Pot 2	Pot 3
For 'established technologies' including onshore wind and solar power projects	For 'less-established technologies' including offshore wind and biomass with combined heat and power	For biomass conversions
The Department expects a high number of projects to seek a contract for difference and intends to set its budget or deployment limit at a level lower than required to meet fully the demand to enable competition	The Department may set its budget at a level approximately equivalent to demand, so that price competition only occurs if demand is high	The Department is still considering whether it can drive effective competition

Source: Department of Energy & Climate Change

Appendix One

Our audit approach

1 In May 2014, the Department of Energy & Climate Change (the Department) signed early contracts for difference for eight renewable electricity projects under its Final Investment Decision enabling for Renewables (FIDeR) scheme. We examined the rationale for this scheme and the risk to value for money from these contracts. We reviewed the Department's:

- business case for the scheme;
- budget setting for these contracts;
- process for selecting these contracts;
- setting of strike prices for these contracts; and
- risks to value for money.

2 Our evaluation criteria addressed the Department's rationale for the FIDeR scheme, whether it was clearly defined and informed by robust evidence and supported through its evaluation criteria, and whether the outturn from early contract awards under the scheme met the Department's purposes and the implications for value for money.

3 Our audit approach is summarised in **Figure 11** overleaf. Our evidence base is described in Appendix Two.

Figure 11
Our audit approach

The Department's objective

The Department is aiming to provide secure, low carbon and affordable energy for consumers.

How this will be achieved

The Department is reforming the schemes it runs to encourage investment in new renewable electricity generation. Before these reforms are complete, the Department gave early contracts to certain renewable electricity projects to address the risk that investors would delay viable projects until reforms have been completed.

Our study

The study examined the rationale for the FIDeR scheme and the value for money of these early contracts.

Our evaluative criteria

Whether the Department's rationale for the scheme was clearly defined and informed by a robust business case and supported through its evaluation criteria for selecting projects for early contracts.

How well the scheme has met the Department's objectives and so achieved good value for money for consumers.

Our evidence

(see Appendix Two for details)

We have reviewed:

- the Department's business cases, and supporting analysis and modelling;
- the Department's budget options analysis;
- internal and external reviews of the scheme.

We have reviewed:

- the Department's selection criteria and other process documents;
- applicants' submissions;
- the Department's assessments and scoring;
- the Department's affordability modelling.

We have undertaken:

- stakeholder interviews;
- a review of the Department's strike price setting methodology and calculation models;
- a review of draft and final contracts.

Our conclusions

Early contracts for renewables have helped industry confidence in the near term and the projects they support can make a significant contribution to meeting the UK's 2020 renewable energy target. The contracts themselves are designed to offer better value for money than the Renewables Obligation they replace. But the contracts have been awarded without price competition and with administratively set strike prices which may provide higher returns than needed to secure investment. We are not convinced that it was essential to award so much consumer support to early contracts in order to meet the 2020 renewables target. Awarding so many early contracts of this scale in this way has limited the Department's opportunity to secure better value for money through competition under the full regime which will start to award contracts in December of this year. The value from the early contracts is in part the learning they can deliver to help transition towards a competitive regime for contracts for difference but this value will be lost if the Department does not get competition into place while a substantial part of the funding remains available.

Appendix Two

Our evidence base

1 We reached our independent conclusions on rationale for the early contracts awarded under the Final Investment Decision enabling Renewables scheme and the risks to value for money, after analysing evidence collected between March and May 2014.

2 We considered:

- whether the rationale was clearly defined and informed by robust evidence;
- whether the design and outcome of the scheme's selection process met the Department's objectives and achieved good value for money for consumers; and
- whether the Department appropriately considered implications for value for money in the contract terms and strike prices.

Our audit approach is outlined in Appendix One.

3 We assessed whether the rationale was clearly defined and informed by robust evidence:

- We reviewed published impact assessments and unpublished business cases for the scheme, and supporting evidence and analysis conducted by the Department, such as the Department modelling of deployment using its Dynamic Dispatch Model.
- We examined governance documents for the scheme including the findings of internal scrutiny by the Department and external reviews conducted by the Major Projects Authority.

4 We considered whether the design and outcome of the scheme's selection process met the Department's objectives and achieved good value for money for consumers:

- We reviewed the Department's qualification, evaluation and down-selection process, examining the criteria used by the Department, the resources it deployed and its assessments of applicants' submissions.
- We also reviewed the Department's analysis of affordability and the application of its affordability down-selection rules.
- We interviewed the following industry stakeholders to understand their views on the scheme and its operation:
  - Dong Energy
  - Repsol
  - GDF Suez
  - Eggborough Power Limited
  - Mainstream
  - SSE
  - Northfield Power
  - Ecotricity
  - RWE
  - MGT Power
  - Siemens
  - Statkraft
- We examined project planning documents to understand the changes in the Department's timetable and the impact on the potential for saving investment delays.

5 We considered whether the Department appropriately considered implications for value for money in the contract terms and strike prices for these contracts:

- We reviewed draft and final contracts to understand the implications for public value in the contract terms.
- We examined the Department's methodology for deriving strike prices, and its model for calculating the strike price to align with Renewables Obligation bands, including assumptions on hurdle rates.
- We examined the Department's proposals for allocating contracts under the main Contracts for Difference scheme, the potential for price competition, and the implications for the value for money of early contracts.

Report by the Comptroller and Auditor General

Early contracts for renewable electricity

HC 172 Session 2014-15

ISBN 9781904219255

Ordered by the House of Commons to be printed on 26 June 2014

CORRECTION

Figure 7 (page 31) of the report was produced in error.

There are two rows labelled 'Offshore wind'. The first of these rows should be labelled 'Onshore wind'.

Please see the corrected figure overleaf:

Figure 7

Operational and planned electricity generation capacity from offshore wind, onshore wind and biomass plants in April 2014

There should be sufficient generation capacity in the pipeline to meet the 2020 renewables target

		Projects with planning consent				Projects awaiting planning consent			
Technology (MW)	Operational	Under construction	Awaiting construction	Total capacity with planning consent or operational	Supported through FIDeR	Capacity awaiting planning consent	Supported through FIDeR	Total capacity operational or in the planning pipeline	Deployment in 2020: EMR Delivery Plan, December 2013 (incl small scale generation)
Onshore wind	7,406	1,539	5,226	14,170	0	6,432	0	20,603	11,700 – 14,100
Offshore wind	3,969	1,401	4,152	9,522	1,066	12,338	2,118	21,860	8,100 – 15,000
Biomass	3,136	268	2,217	5,621	1,364	299	0	5,919	2,500 – 4,600
Total for onshore wind, offshore wind and Biomass	14,511	3,208	11,594	29,313	2,430	19,069	2,118	48,381	22,300 – 33,700 25,600 (deployment in Electricity Market Reform Delivery Plan reference case)

Notes

1 We have taken deployment ranges in 2020 from the Department's modelling for its Electricitiy Market Reform final delivery plan, December 2013. The single total is from the reference case developed for this modelling which is Scenario 1 in the delivery plan.

2 Other data is taken from the Department's Renewables Energy Planning Database, Progress datasheet, May 2014.

3 Biomass includes biomass conversion and biomass combined heat and power.

4 Not all of this capacity will be installed as projects awaiting construction may not be built and projects may not receive planning consent. The rate of attrition will vary from technology to technology.

5 Planning pipelines do not take into account sensitivities such as the possible impact of policy developments or changes in financial support rates.

6 Data may not sum due to rounding.

Source: Department of Energy & Climate Change

Paragraph 3.11 (page 33) the last sentence of 3.11 should end with 'such as carbon capture and storage.' The text: 'stated that it will… within the Levy Control Framework.' Should be deleted, as it is repeated correctly at the end of paragraph 3.12.

Please see the incorrect paragraph below:

3.11 By using a high proportion of the latest estimates of the available Levy Control Framework budget, early contracts may reduce industry confidence in getting support later in the decade. Stakeholders we spoke to noted that the constrained funds available for other renewable contracts for difference increased the allocation risk for future projects. Assuming these projects commission at their target commissioning date and at their full capacity, they will cost £4 billion to 2020-21, 58 per cent of the £6.9 billion we estimate is available for all renewable contracts for difference. In 2020-21, these projects will cost £1.2 billion, 65 per cent of the £1.8 billion available in that year (**Figure 8** overleaf).[6] The amount of funding available for new contracts will depend on the Department's controls on spending on other schemes. For example, the cost of the Renewables Obligation could increase if large numbers of renewable generation projects seek to accredit before it closes in 2017. The budget available for contracts for difference for renewables also depends on the strike prices agreed and the actual commissioning date for non-renewable projects, such as carbon capture and storage~~, stated that it will maintain the 'buying power' of the Levy Control Framework. To do this, it is increasing its Levy Control Framework budget by around £170 million in 2020-21 (2013-14 prices), but is not altering the overall cap. So it is reducing the contingency available to absorb other cost increases within the Levy Control Framework~~.

Please see the corrected paragraph below:

3.11 By using a high proportion of the latest estimates of the available Levy Control Framework budget, early contracts may reduce industry confidence in getting support later in the decade. Stakeholders we spoke to noted that the constrained funds available for other renewable contracts for difference increased the allocation risk for future projects. Assuming these projects commission at their target commissioning date and at their full capacity, they will cost £4 billion to 2020-21, 58 per cent of the £6.9 billion we estimate is available for all renewable contracts for difference. In 2020-21, these projects will cost £1.2 billion, 65 per cent of the £1.8 billion available in that year (**Figure 8** overleaf).[6] The amount of funding available for new contracts will depend on the Department's controls on spending on other schemes. For example, the cost of the Renewables Obligation could increase if large numbers of renewable generation projects seek to accredit before it closes in 2017. The budget available for contracts for difference for renewables also depends on the strike prices agreed and the actual commissioning date for non-renewable projects, such as carbon capture and storage.

6 Cost data are in 2013-14 prices. The Department considers these eight FIDeR projects may deliver less than the full capacity stated by developers and could commission later than target commissioning dates. On the basis of its adjusted estimates of capacity and commissioning dates, the Department's central estimate of the cost of these contracts between 2015-16 and 2020-21 is £3.2 billion (undiscounted), 47 per cent of the available funds. In 2020-21, the Department's central estimate is that they will cost £1 billion, 57 per cent of the available funds in that year.

Please see the following paragraph with the repeated wording:

3.12 At the Budget 2014, the government decided to cap the carbon price floor from 2016-17 to 2019-20. The higher the carbon price floor, the higher the tax paid on fossil fuels used for electricity generation. Capping it means that wholesale electricity prices are lower than if the carbon price had been allowed to rise in line with original plans. This is turn means difference payments under contracts for difference are higher. This has increased the risk that the Department may not be able to allocate enough contracts for difference to support investment to meet the renewables target within the Levy Control Framework caps. Using the Department's data, we estimate that capping the carbon price floor will add £225 million to the cost of these early contracts between 2016-17 and 2020-21, of which around £85 million is in 2020-21. The Department has stated that it will maintain the 'buying power' of the Levy Control Framework. To do this, it is increasing its Levy Control Framework budget by around £170 million in 2020-21 (2013-14 prices), but is not altering the overall cap. So it is reducing the contingency available to absorb other cost increases within the Levy Control Framework.

Appendix One, paragraph 1 (page 43) 'In May 2013' should read 'In May 2014'

Please see the corrected paragraph below:

1 In May 2014, the Department of Energy & Climate Change (the Department) signed early contracts for difference for eight renewable electricity projects under its Final Investment Decision enabling for Renewables (FIDeR) scheme. We examined the rationale for this scheme and the risk to value for money from these contracts. We reviewed the Department's:

- business case for the scheme;
- budget setting for these contracts;
- process for selecting these contracts;
- setting of strike prices for these contracts; and
- risks to value for money.